AYURVEDIC COOKING

Nourish Your Body and Soul with Ancient Wisdom

By: Swati

CONTENTS

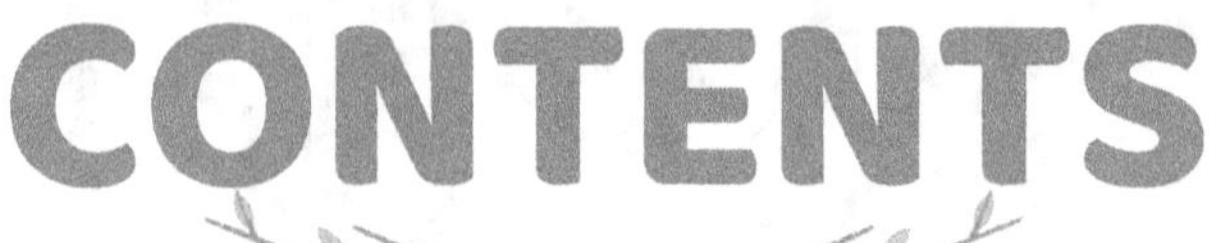

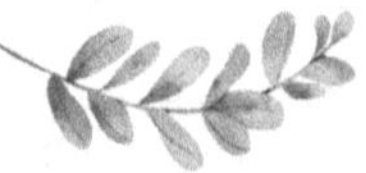

Introduction

Welcome to the world of Ayurvedic cooking, where food is not just sustenance but a powerful tool for healing and balance

Ayurveda, the ancient Indian system of medicine, views food as medicine and emphasizes the importance of eating according to your body type and the seasons

In this book, we'll explore the principles of Ayurvedic cooking and learn how to create delicious and nutritious meals that promote health and well-being

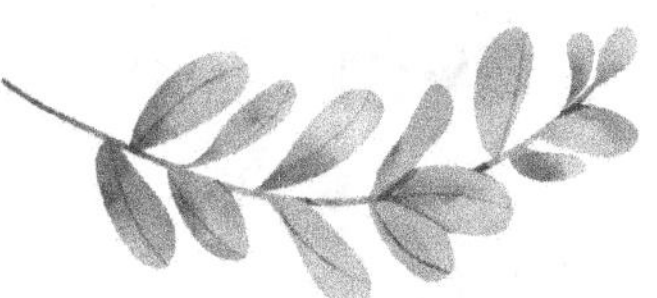

Chapter 1
The Fundamentals of Ayurvedic Cooking

-<u>Understanding the Doshas</u>: Learn about Vata, Pitta, and Kapha – the three doshas that govern our bodies and how they influence our dietary needs

- <u>The Six Tastes</u>: Explore the six tastes – sweet, sour, salty, bitter, pungent, and astringent and how incorporating all of them into your meals can help balance your doshas

- <u>Eating with the Seasons</u>: Discover how eating seasonally can support your body's natural rhythms and promote optimal health

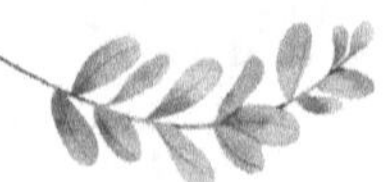

Chapter 2
Ayurvedic Ingredients and Spices

- <u>Staple Foods</u>: **Learn about the staple foods in Ayurvedic cooking including grains, legumes, vegetables, fruits, nuts, and seeds**

- <u>Healing Spices</u>: **Explore the medicinal properties of common Ayurvedic spices such as turmeric, ginger, cumin, coriander, and fenugreek, and how to use them in your cooking**

- <u>Ghee and Oils</u>: **Understand the importance of ghee (clarified butter) and other oils in Ayurvedic cooking and how to choose the right ones for your constitution**

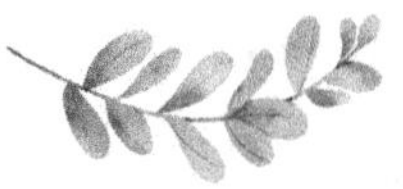

Chapter 3
Cooking Methods and Techniques

- **Sattvic Cooking:** Discover the principles of Sattvic cooking, which emphasises purity, simplicity, and mindfulness in food preparation

- **Ayurvedic Cooking Techniques:** Learn about cooking methods such as sautéing, steaming, boiling, and baking, and how to use them to preserve the nutritional value of your ingredients

- **Food Combining:** Understand the principles of food combining in Ayurveda and how it can support digestion and nutrient absorption

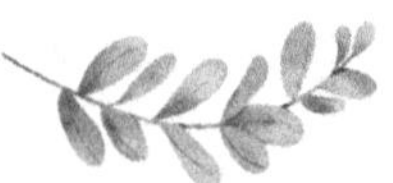

Chapter 4
Ayurvedic Meal Planning

- <u>Building Balanced Meals:</u> **Learn how to create balanced meals that include all six tastes and are tailored to your unique dosha constitution**

- <u>Daily Routines:</u> **Explore the importance of establishing daily routines in Ayurveda, including meal times, exercise, meditation, and sleep, and how they contribute to overall well-being**

- <u>Ayurvedic Cleanses:</u> **Discover gentle Ayurvedic cleanses and detoxification practices to rejuvenate your body and mind**

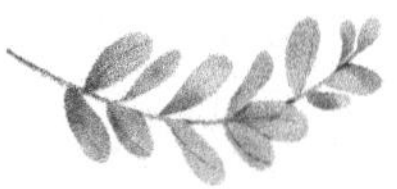

Chapter 5
Ayurvedic Recipes

- <u>Breakfast</u>:
Start your day with nourishing breakfast recipes such as spiced oatmeal, quinoa porridge, and fruit smoothies

- <u>Lunch and Dinner</u>:
Enjoy flavorful lunch and dinner recipes including lentil dal, vegetable curry, kitchari, and stuffed bell peppers

- <u>Snacks and Desserts</u>:
Indulge in healthy snacks and desserts like roasted chickpeas, almond date balls, and chai-spiced rice pudding

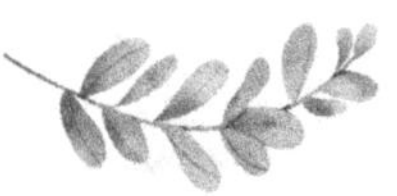

Chapter 6
Special Diets and Adaptations

- <u>Ayurveda for Vegetarians and Vegans:</u>
Discover how to adapt Ayurvedic principles to vegetarian and vegan diets while still meeting your nutritional needs

- <u>Ayurveda for Weight Management:</u>
Learn about Ayurvedic strategies for maintaining a healthy weight, including mindful eating, portion control, and balancing your doshas

- <u>Ayurveda for Healing:</u> Explore how Ayurvedic cooking can support healing from specific health conditions such as digestive disorders, inflammation, and stress

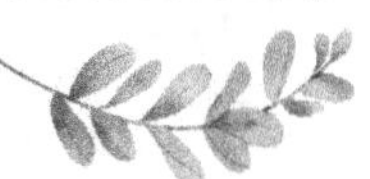

Conclusion

In Ayurvedic cooking, food is more than just sustenance – it's a pathway to health, vitality, and balance

By understanding the principles of Ayurveda and incorporating them into your cooking, you can nourish your body, mind, and soul and cultivate a deeper connection to yourself and the world around you

Embrace the wisdom of Ayurveda and let it guide you on your journey to vibrant health and well-being

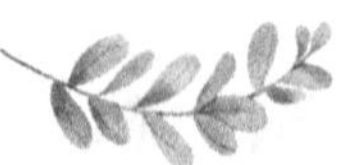

Chapter 1
The Fundamentals of Ayurvedic Cooking

Ayurvedic cooking is rooted in the ancient Indian system of medicine known as Ayurveda, which views food as a powerful tool for healing and balance

At the core of Ayurvedic cooking are the principles of harmony, balance, and individualised nutrition

In this chapter, we'll explore the fundamentals of Ayurvedic cooking, including the three doshas, the six tastes, and the importance of eating with the seasons

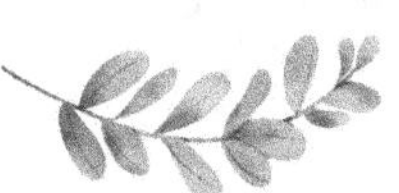

Chapter 1
The Fundamentals of Ayurvedic Cooking

Understanding the Doshas

Ayurveda recognises three fundamental energies or doshas – Vata, Pitta, and Kapha – that govern our bodies and minds. Each person has a unique combination of these doshas, which influences their physical, mental, and emotional characteristics. Understanding your dominant dosha(s) is essential for tailoring your diet to promote balance and well-being

- Vata: Associated with the elements of air and ether, Vata governs movement, creativity, and communication. A balanced Vata diet includes warm, grounding foods that provide nourishment and stability
- Pitta: Linked to the elements of fire and water, Pitta governs digestion, metabolism, and intellect. A balanced Pitta diet includes cooling, soothing foods that help maintain a calm and balanced mind
- Kapha: Rooted in the elements of earth and water, Kapha governs structure, stability, and growth. A balanced Kapha diet includes light, stimulating foods that support digestion and energy levels

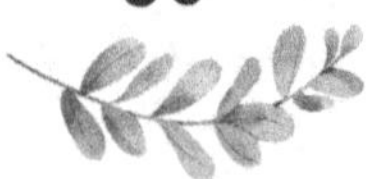

Chapter 1
The Fundamentals of Ayurvedic Cooking

The Six Tastes

Ayurveda recognises six tastes – sweet, sour, salty, bitter, pungent, and astringent – each of which plays a unique role in balancing the doshas and promoting overall health. Including all six tastes in your meals ensures that you receive a wide range of nutrients and flavors, supporting optimal digestion and satisfaction

- Sweet: Nourishing and grounding, sweet foods include grains, root vegetables, fruits, and natural sweeteners like honey and maple syrup.
- Sour: Refreshing and cleansing, sour foods include citrus fruits, yogurt, fermented foods, and vinegar.
- Salty: Hydrating and stimulating, salty foods include sea salt, seaweed, and naturally salty foods like celery and olives
- Bitter: Detoxifying and cooling, bitter foods include leafy greens, bitter gourds, turmeric, and bitter herbs like dandelion and neem
- Pungent: Warming and invigorating, pungent foods include garlic, onions, ginger, chili peppers, and spices like black pepper and mustard seeds
- Astringent: Balancing and drying, astringent foods include beans, lentils, green tea, and certain fruits like pomegranates and cranberries

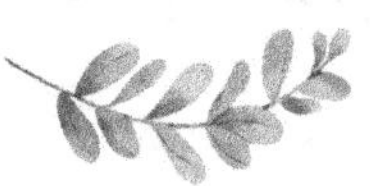

Chapter 1
The Fundamentals of Ayurvedic Cooking

Eating with the Seasons

In Ayurveda, eating with the seasons is considered essential for maintaining balance and harmony with nature. Each season has its own unique qualities that influence our bodies and minds, and adjusting our diet accordingly can help us stay healthy and resilient throughout the year

- Spring: As the weather warms and the earth awakens, focus on light, cleansing foods like leafy greens, sprouts, and bitter herbs to support detoxification and renewal

- Summer: Stay cool and hydrated with juicy fruits, fresh vegetables, and cooling herbs like mint and cilantro. Avoid heavy, oily foods and opt for lighter, refreshing meals

- Autumn: As temperatures begin to cool and the days shorten, incorporate warm, grounding foods like root vegetables, whole grains, and hearty soups to nourish and comfort the body

- Winter: Keep warm and nourished during the cold winter months with hearty stews, cooked grains, and nourishing spices like cinnamon, ginger, and cloves. Focus on building strength and resilience to withstand the challenges of winter

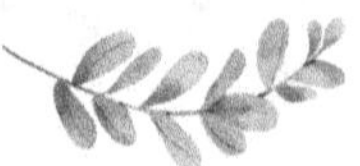

Chapter 1
The Fundamentals of Ayurvedic Cooking

By understanding the doshas, incorporating the six tastes, and eating with the seasons, you can cultivate a balanced and harmonious approach to Ayurvedic cooking that supports your health and well-being on every level.

In the following chapters, we'll delve deeper into Ayurvedic ingredients, cooking methods, and recipes to help you harness the healing power of food and transform your relationship with eating.

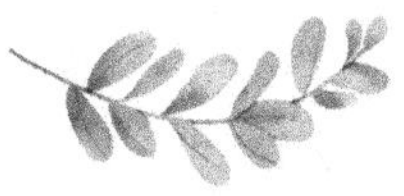

Chapter 2
Ayurvedic Ingredients and Spices

Ayurvedic cooking is characterized by the use of wholesome, natural ingredients and aromatic spices that not only add flavor to dishes but also promote health and well-being

In this chapter, we'll explore the staple foods, healing spices, and nourishing oils used in Ayurvedic cuisine

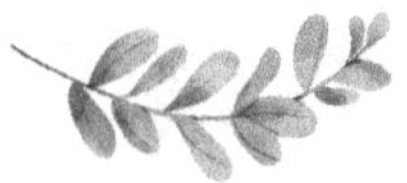

Chapter 2
Ayurvedic Ingredients and Spices

Staple Foods

Ayurvedic cooking emphasises the importance of whole, unprocessed foods that are nourishing and easy to digest. Here are some staple foods commonly used in Ayurvedic cuisine

- Grains: Whole grains like rice, quinoa, millet, barley, and oats are a staple in Ayurvedic cooking. They provide energy, fiber, and essential nutrients, and can be prepared in a variety of ways

- Legumes: Lentils, beans, and split peas are rich in protein, fiber, and minerals, making them an important source of plant-based protein in Ayurvedic cuisine. They're also easy to digest when properly cooked and seasoned

- Vegetables: Fresh, seasonal vegetables are the foundation of Ayurvedic meals, providing a wide range of vitamins, minerals, and phytonutrients. Leafy greens, root vegetables, cruciferous vegetables, and squashes are all commonly used

- Fruits: Sweet, juicy fruits like apples, pears, berries, and citrus fruits are enjoyed in moderation in Ayurvedic cooking. They provide natural sweetness and hydration, and can be eaten fresh or cooked

- Nuts and Seeds: Almonds, walnuts, sesame seeds, sunflower seeds, and pumpkin seeds are rich in healthy fats, protein, and minerals. They're often used as toppings, garnishes, or in homemade nut milks and seed butters

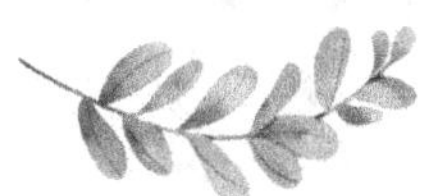

Chapter 2
Ayurvedic Ingredients and Spices

Healing Spices

Spices play a central role in Ayurvedic cooking, not only for their flavor-enhancing properties but also for their medicinal benefits. Here are some common healing spices used in Ayurvedic cuisine

- Turmeric: Known for its vibrant yellow color and anti-inflammatory properties, turmeric is a staple in Ayurvedic cooking. It's often used in curries, soups, and rice dishes to add flavor and color

- Ginger: Spicy and warming, ginger is prized for its digestive properties and ability to relieve nausea and indigestion. It can be used fresh or dried in teas, soups, stir-fries, and baked goods

- Cumin: Earthy and aromatic, cumin aids digestion, reduces bloating, and enhances the flavor of dishes. It's commonly used in dals, spice blends, and vegetable dishes

- Coriander: Mild and citrusy, coriander balances the flavors of spicy dishes and aids digestion. Both the seeds and fresh leaves (cilantro) are used in Ayurvedic cooking

- Fenugreek: Bitter and aromatic, fenugreek seeds are believed to improve digestion, regulate blood sugar levels, and support lactation in nursing mothers. They're often used in spice blends and vegetable dishes

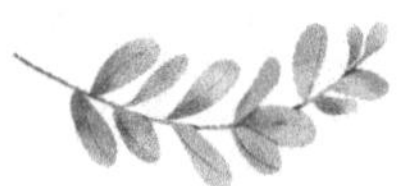

Chapter 2
Ayurvedic Ingredients and Spices

Ghee and Oils

Ghee, or clarified butter, is a revered ingredient in Ayurvedic cooking prized for its rich flavor and medicinal properties. Made by simmering butter and removing the milk solids, ghee is lactose-free and has a high smoke point, making it suitable for cooking at high temperatures

In addition to ghee, Ayurvedic cooking also incorporates a variety of nourishing oils such as sesame oil, coconut oil, and mustard oil, each with its own unique flavor and health benefits

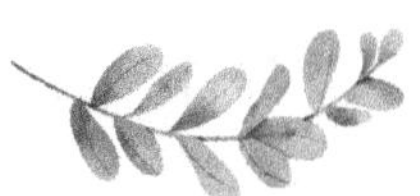

Chapter 2
Ayurvedic Ingredients and Spices

By incorporating these wholesome ingredients and healing spices into your cooking, you can create delicious and nourishing meals that support your health and well-being according to the principles of Ayurveda. In the following chapters, we'll explore Ayurvedic cooking techniques, meal planning, and recipes to help you harness the full potential of these ingredients and spices

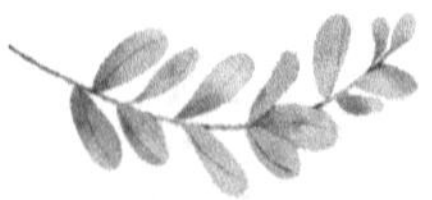

Chapter 3
Ayurvedic Cooking Methods and Techniques

Ayurvedic cooking emphasises the use of gentle, nourishing cooking methods that preserve the natural flavors and nutrients of ingredients while promoting easy digestion and assimilation

In this chapter, we'll explore the cooking methods and techniques commonly used in Ayurvedic cuisine

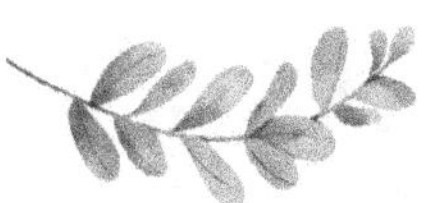

Chapter 3
Ayurvedic Cooking Methods and Techniques

Sattvic Cooking:

At the heart of Ayurvedic cooking is the concept of Sattvic food, which is pure, light, and balanced

Sattvic cooking focuses on using fresh, seasonal ingredients and simple preparation methods to create meals that are nourishing for the body, mind, and spirit. Some key principles of Sattvic cooking include:

- Using fresh, organic ingredients whenever possible

- Cooking with love and mindfulness

- Avoiding processed foods, additives, and preservatives

- Balancing the six tastes (sweet, sour, salty, bitter, pungent, and astringent) in each meal

- Cooking with awareness of the seasons and their influence on our bodies

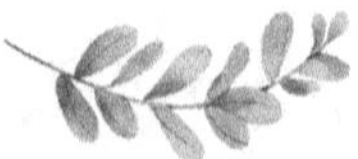

Chapter 3
Ayurvedic Cooking Methods and Techniques

Ayurvedic Cooking Techniques

Ayurvedic cooking employs a variety of cooking techniques that are designed to enhance the flavor and digestibility of food while preserving its nutritional value. Here are some common Ayurvedic cooking techniques:

- **Sautéing:** Sautéing involves cooking ingredients in a small amount of ghee or oil over medium heat until they are lightly browned and aromatic. This technique is often used to cook vegetables, spices, and aromatics at the beginning of a recipe to build flavor

- **Steaming:** Steaming involves cooking food over boiling water in a covered pot or steamer basket. This gentle cooking method helps to retain the natural moisture and nutrients of ingredients while preserving their color and texture. Steaming is commonly used for vegetables, grains, and dumplings

- **Boiling:** Boiling involves cooking ingredients in a large amount of water until they are tender and cooked through. This method is often used for cooking grains, legumes, and soups, and can help to soften tough or fibrous ingredients

- **Baking:** Baking involves cooking food in an oven at a moderate temperature until it is cooked through and golden brown. This dry heat cooking method is commonly used for baking bread, cakes, cookies, and savory dishes like casseroles and roasted vegetables

- **Stir-frying:** Stir-frying involves cooking ingredients in a small amount of oil over high heat while continuously stirring or tossing them in the pan. This quick cooking method helps to preserve the natural crunch and color of ingredients while infusing them with flavor from the spices and aromatics

- **Pressure cooking:** Pressure cooking involves cooking food in a sealed pot under high pressure, which increases the temperature and reduces the cooking time. This method is particularly useful for cooking grains, legumes, and tough cuts of meat, and helps to retain the natural flavors and nutrients of ingredients

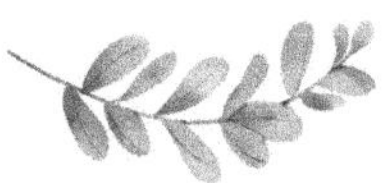

Chapter 3
Ayurvedic Cooking Methods and Techniques

Food Combining

In Ayurvedic cooking, food combining plays a crucial role in promoting optimal digestion and nutrient absorption
Certain food combinations are believed to support digestion and balance the doshas, while others may hinder digestion and lead to discomfort or imbalance

Some basic principles of food combining in Ayurveda include:

- Eating fruits separately from other foods, preferably on an empty stomach or as a snack between meals
- Avoiding combining milk with sour or salty foods, as it may cause digestive issues
- Pairing grains with vegetables and legumes for a balanced meal that provides all essential nutrients
- Using spices and herbs to aid digestion and enhance the flavor of dishes

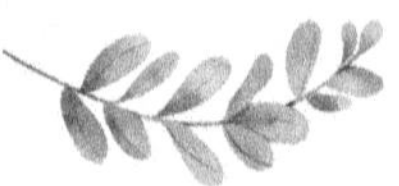

Chapter 3
Ayurvedic Cooking Methods and Techniques

By mastering these Ayurvedic cooking methods and techniques, you can create nourishing and delicious meals that support your health and well-being on every level

In the following chapters, we'll explore Ayurvedic meal planning, recipes, and special diets to help you incorporate these principles into your daily life and experience the transformative power of Ayurvedic cuisine

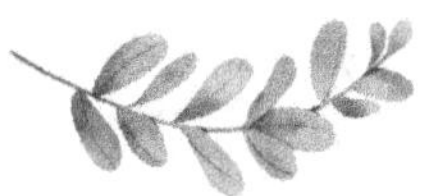

Chapter 4
Ayurvedic Meal Planning

Ayurvedic meal planning is centered around creating balanced, nourishing meals that support your unique constitution and promote health and well-being

In this chapter, we'll explore the principles of Ayurvedic meal planning, including building balanced meals, establishing daily routines, and incorporating Ayurvedic cleanses

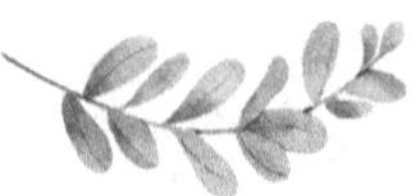

Chapter 4
Ayurvedic Meal Planning

Building Balanced Meals

Ayurvedic meal planning emphasises the importance of including all six tastes (sweet, sour, salty, bitter, pungent, and astringent) in each meal to ensure that you receive a wide range of nutrients and flavors.

Here's a guide to building balanced Ayurvedic meals

1. **Start with a Base:** Choose a whole grain or starchy vegetable as the foundation of your meal, such as rice, quinoa, millet, sweet potatoes, or squash

2. **Add Protein:** Include a source of protein to help you feel satisfied and support muscle repair and growth. Good options include lentils, beans, tofu, tempeh, nuts, seeds, and dairy products (if tolerated)

3. **Incorporate Vegetables:** Fill half of your plate with a variety of colorful vegetables, including leafy greens, cruciferous vegetables, root vegetables, and seasonal produce

4. **Include Healthy Fats:** Add a small amount of healthy fats to your meal to support brain health, hormone production, and nutrient absorption. Good options include ghee, olive oil, avocado, nuts, and seeds

5. **Season with Spices:** Use Ayurvedic spices to enhance the flavor and digestibility of your meals. Experiment with warming spices like ginger, turmeric, cumin, coriander, and fennel to balance your doshas and promote optimal digestion

6. **Enjoy Mindfully:** Sit down to eat in a calm, relaxed environment, and chew your food slowly and thoroughly to aid digestion and enhance nutrient absorption

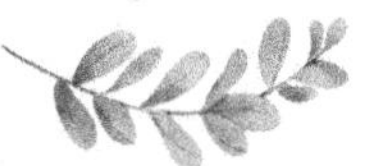

Chapter 4
Ayurvedic Meal Planning

Establishing Daily Routines

In Ayurveda, establishing daily routines, or dinacharya, is considered essential for maintaining balance and promoting health and well-being

Here are some key daily routines to incorporate into your life:

- **Rise with the Sun:** Wake up early in the morning, preferably before sunrise, to align with the natural rhythms of nature and maximize your energy and vitality
- **Practice Self-Care:** Take time each day to care for your body, mind, and spirit through practices like meditation, yoga, self-massage (abhyanga), and deep breathing exercises
- **Eat Regular Meals:** Establish regular meal times and try to eat your meals at roughly the same times each day to support digestion and stabilize your energy levels
- **Move Your Body:** Incorporate regular exercise into your daily routine to strengthen your body, improve circulation, and promote overall health and vitality
- **Wind Down at Night:** Create a calming bedtime routine to help you relax and prepare for restful sleep. Avoid stimulating activities like screen time and heavy meals close to bedtime

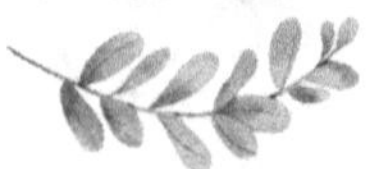

Chapter 4
Ayurvedic Meal Planning

Ayurvedic Cleanses

Ayurvedic cleanses, or kitchari cleanses, are gentle detoxification practices designed to support the body's natural detoxification processes and promote balance and well-being

A typical kitchari cleanse involves eating a simple diet of kitchari – a nourishing blend of rice, lentils, vegetables, and spices – for a period of three to seven days, along with herbal teas and digestive tonics

During the cleanse, you'll eliminate caffeine, alcohol, processed foods, and other potential toxins from your diet, allowing your body to reset and rejuvenate

Chapter 4
Ayurvedic Meal Planning

By incorporating these principles of Ayurvedic meal planning, daily routines, and cleanses into your life, you can nourish your body, mind, and spirit and cultivate a deeper sense of health and well-being

In the following chapters, we'll explore Ayurvedic recipes and special diets to help you put these principles into practice and experience the transformative power of Ayurvedic cuisine

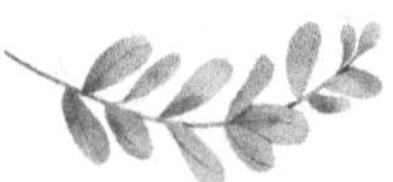

Chapter 5
Ayurvedic Recipes

In this chapter, we'll explore a variety of delicious and nourishing Ayurvedic recipes that are designed to support your health and well-being according to the principles of Ayurveda

From breakfast to dinner, and even snacks and desserts, these recipes are filled with wholesome ingredients and aromatic spices that will delight your senses and nourish your body

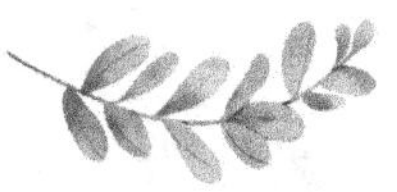

Chapter 5
Ayurvedic Recipes

Breakfast Recipes

1. **Spiced Oatmeal:** Cook rolled oats with water or milk (dairy or plant-based) and add a pinch of cinnamon, cardamom, and ginger. Top with chopped nuts, seeds, and fresh fruit for added flavor and texture

2. **Quinoa Porridge:** Cook quinoa with milk (dairy or plant-based) and sweeten with a touch of honey or maple syrup. Add diced apples, raisins, and a sprinkle of cinnamon for a warming and nourishing breakfast

3. **Fruit Smoothie:** Blend together your favorite fruits (such as bananas, berries, mangoes, or peaches) with yogurt or coconut milk, a handful of spinach or kale, and a dash of honey or dates for sweetness. Add a pinch of ginger or turmeric for an extra boost of flavor and health benefits

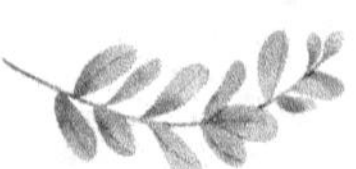

Chapter 5
Ayurvedic Recipes

Lunch and Dinner Recipes

1. **Lentil Dal:** Cook lentils with water, spices (such as cumin, coriander, turmeric, and ginger), and diced vegetables (such as onions, tomatoes, carrots, and spinach). Serve over rice or quinoa for a hearty and satisfying meal

2. **Vegetable Curry:** Sauté onions, garlic, and ginger in ghee or oil, then add diced vegetables (such as potatoes, cauliflower, bell peppers, and peas) and simmer in a flavorful curry sauce made with coconut milk and spices (such as curry powder, turmeric, cumin, and coriander)

3. **Kitchari:** Cook a simple kitchari by simmering rice, lentils, vegetables (such as carrots, zucchini, and spinach), and spices (such as cumin, turmeric, and coriander) in water or broth until tender. Serve hot with a dollop of ghee for a comforting and nourishing meal

Chapter 5
Ayurvedic Recipes

Snacks and Desserts

1. **Roasted Chickpeas:** Toss cooked chickpeas with olive oil and spices (such as cumin, paprika, and garlic powder) and roast in the oven until crispy. Enjoy as a crunchy and satisfying snack

2. **Almond Date Balls:** Blend together dates, almonds, coconut flakes, and a pinch of cinnamon in a food processor until smooth. Roll into balls and coat in additional coconut flakes for a sweet and energizing treat

3. **Chai-Spiced Rice Pudding:** Cook rice with milk (dairy or plant-based) and sweeten with honey or maple syrup. Add warming spices like cinnamon, cardamom, cloves, and ginger for a fragrant and comforting dessert

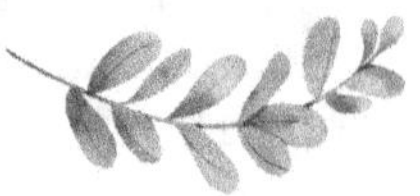

Chapter 5
Ayurvedic Recipes

These Ayurvedic recipes are just a starting point for incorporating the principles of Ayurveda into your cooking

Feel free to experiment with different ingredients, spices, and flavor combinations to create meals that suit your tastes and nourish your body according to your unique constitution

In the next chapter, we'll explore special diets and adaptations for vegetarian, vegan, and weight management purposes

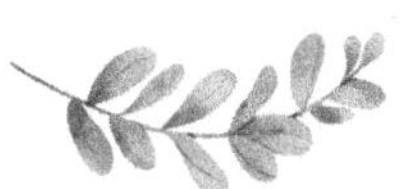

Chapter 6
Special Diets and Adaptations

Ayurveda recognizes that each person is unique, with individual dietary needs and preferences

Whether you're following a vegetarian or vegan diet, looking to manage your weight, or seeking to address specific health concerns, Ayurvedic cooking offers a variety of adaptations and special diets to support your goals

In this chapter, we'll explore how to tailor Ayurvedic principles to different dietary preferences and health considerations

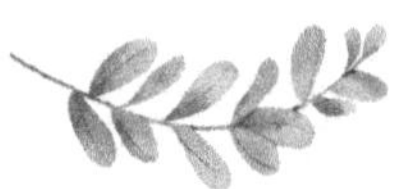

Chapter 6
Special Diets and Adaptations

Ayurveda for Vegetarians and Vegans

Many aspects of Ayurvedic cooking naturally align with vegetarian and vegan diets, which prioritize plant-based foods and abstain from animal products

Here are some tips for adapting Ayurvedic cooking to vegetarian and vegan lifestyles

- **Emphasize Plant-Based Proteins:** Include plenty of beans, lentils, tofu, tempeh, nuts, and seeds in your meals to ensure you're getting enough protein

- **Use Dairy Alternatives:** Substitute dairy products like milk, yogurt, and ghee with plant-based alternatives such as almond milk, coconut yogurt, and coconut oil

- **Focus on Whole Foods:** Choose whole, unprocessed plant foods like fruits, vegetables, whole grains, and legumes to maximize the nutritional value of your meals

- **Experiment with Ayurvedic Spices:** Incorporate Ayurvedic spices like turmeric, ginger, cumin, coriander, and fenugreek into your cooking to add flavor and health benefits

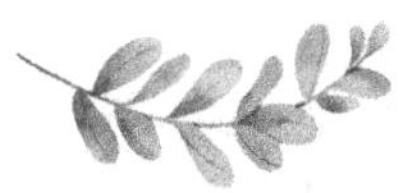

Chapter 6
Special Diets and Adaptations

Ayurveda for Weight Management

Ayurveda offers a holistic approach to weight management that focuses on balancing the doshas, supporting digestion, and promoting overall health and well-being

Here are some Ayurvedic strategies for maintaining a healthy weight

- Eat Mindfully: Practice mindful eating by paying attention to hunger and fullness cues, savoring each bite, and avoiding distractions while eating

- Choose Whole Foods: Opt for whole, unprocessed foods that are rich in nutrients and fiber, such as fruits, vegetables, whole grains, and lean proteins

- Balance Your Meals: Create balanced meals that include all six tastes – sweet, sour, salty, bitter, pungent, and astringent – to satisfy your palate and prevent cravings

- Avoid Overeating: Eat until you're satisfied, not stuffed, and avoid eating large meals late at night, which can disrupt digestion and lead to weight gain

- Stay Active: Incorporate regular exercise into your daily routine to support metabolism, maintain muscle mass, and promote overall health and vitality

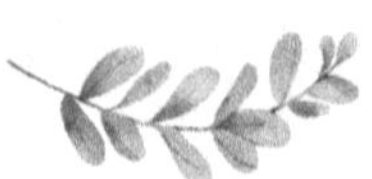

Chapter 6
Special Diets and Adaptations

Ayurveda for Healing

Ayurvedic cooking can also be used to support healing from specific health conditions, such as digestive disorders, inflammation, and stress

Here are some Ayurvedic principles for promoting healing and well-being

- Choose Healing Foods: Include foods that are known for their healing properties, such as ginger, turmeric, garlic, leafy greens, and fermented foods like yogurt and sauerkraut

- Support Digestion: Focus on easy-to-digest foods like soups, stews, cooked vegetables, and well-cooked grains to support digestion and ease digestive discomfort

- Reduce Inflammation: Incorporate anti-inflammatory foods like fatty fish, walnuts, flaxseeds, and dark leafy greens into your diet to help reduce inflammation and support overall health

- Practice Stress Management: Incorporate stress-reducing practices like meditation, yoga, deep breathing exercises, and relaxation techniques to promote balance and well-being

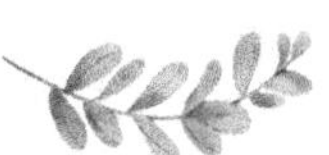

Chapter 6
Special Diets and Adaptations

By adapting Ayurvedic principles to your unique dietary preferences and health goals, you can create a personalized approach to cooking and eating that supports your overall health and well-being

Experiment with different recipes, ingredients, and cooking techniques to discover what works best for you, and remember to listen to your body and honor its needs along the way

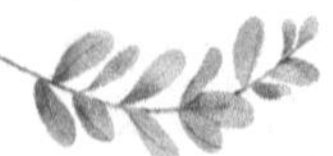

Conclusion:

In conclusion, Ayurvedic cooking offers a holistic approach to nourishing the body, mind, and spirit through food

Rooted in ancient wisdom and guided by the principles of balance, harmony, and individualized nutrition, Ayurvedic cuisine has the power to transform your relationship with eating and promote health and well-being on every level

By understanding the doshas, incorporating the six tastes, and eating with the seasons, you can create balanced and nourishing meals that support your unique constitution and promote optimal health. From wholesome grains and legumes to healing spices and nourishing oils, Ayurvedic cooking celebrates the abundance of nature's bounty and encourages a deep connection to the foods we eat

Through mindful meal planning, daily routines, and special diets and adaptations, Ayurvedic cooking offers a path to healing, transformation, and self-discovery. Whether you're seeking to embrace a vegetarian or vegan lifestyle, manage your weight, or support healing from specific health conditions, Ayurvedic cooking provides a wealth of resources and tools to help you on your journey

As you embark on your Ayurvedic cooking journey, remember to approach it with an open mind, a sense of curiosity, and a spirit of experimentation. Allow yourself to explore new flavors, ingredients, and cooking techniques, and trust in the wisdom of your body to guide you towards foods that nourish and sustain you

Above all, embrace the joy of cooking and eating as a celebration of life and a way to honor the incredible gift of nourishment that sustains

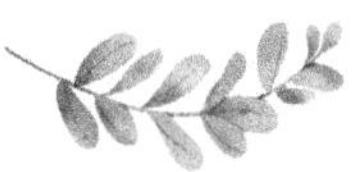

9 798883 028617